POSITIVE SHRINKING

POSITIVE SHRINKING

A Story that Will Change Your

R .... ever

HAY HOUSE

HAY HOUSE

Australia • Canada • Hong Kong • India
South Africa • United Kingdom • United States

First published and distributed in the United Kingdom by:
Hay House UK Ltd, 292B Kensal Rd, London W10 5BE. Tel.: (44) 20 8962 1230;
Fax: (44) 20 8962 1239. www.hayhouse.co.uk

Published and distributed in the United States of America by:
Hay House, Inc., PO Box 5100, Carlsbad, CA 92018-5100. Tel.: (1) 760 431 7695 or
(800) 654 5126; Fax: (1) 760 431 6948 or (800) 650 5115. www.hayhouse.com

Published and distributed in Australia by:
Hay House Australia Ltd, 18/36 Ralph St, Alexandria NSW 2015.
Tel.: (61) 2 9669 4299; Fax: (61) 2 9669 4144. www.hayhouse.com.au

Published and distributed in the Republic of South Africa by:
Hay House SA (Pty), Ltd, PO Box 990, Witkoppen 2068. Tel./Fax: (27) 11 467 8904.
www.hayhouse.co.za

Published and distributed in India by:
Hay House Publishers India, Muskaan Complex, Plot No.3, B-2, Vasant Kunj, New
Delhi – 110 070. Tel.: (91) 11 4176 1620; Fax: (91) 11 4176 1630.
www.hayhouse.co.in

Distributed in Canada by:
Raincoast, 9050 Shaughnessy St, Vancouver, BC V6P 6E5. Tel.: (1) 604 323 7100;
Fax: (1) 604 323 2600

A catalogue record for this book is available from the British Library.

This title was previously self-published by the author, ISBN 978-1-4389-3951-3.

ISBN 978-1-84850-186-7

Printed and bound in the UK by CPI Bookmarque, Croydon, CR0 4TD.

All of the papers used in this product are recyclable, and made from wood grown in
managed, sustainable forests and manufactured at mills certified to ISO 14001 and/
or EMAS.

*This book is dedicated to my great friend
Martin Sterling 1962–2008*

*People only truly die when we forget them.
Anyone who ever met Martin would never be
able to forget him.*

*For Stephen Gately – the world is a lesser place
without you in it and heaven will be a much
brighter place with you there. You were a great
friend, an amazing student and I, like so many
others, will miss your beautiful spirit and angelic
voice. You were the best of the best.*

TABLE OF CONTENTS

(This is the only menu you will find in this book)

PREFACE

WHY THE NEED FOR POSITIVE SHRINKING?

There are thousands of diet books available. They're OK for short-term weight loss, yet in most cases people either return to their pre-diet weight or, more commonly, put on even more – hence the term 'yo-yo dieting'.

Science tells us that maintaining a healthy weight is a simple equation of 'energy in versus energy out'. This is correct, but if it were really that simple why is obesity such a growing problem? *Positive Shrinking* uses established techniques and tools to create a method that means you will be compelled to help yourself reach the goals you desire. It is a lifestyle, not a diet.

WHAT IS POSITIVE SHRINKING?

Positive Shrinking blends methods modelled from sources such as NLP (Neuro Linguistic Programming), TFT (Thought Field Therapy) and other psychological fields to create a simple set of techniques to help you take true control of your eating habits. If I said to you, 'OK, I need to see you gain ten pounds in weight in three weeks,' would you be able to do it? The answer would undoubtedly be 'Yes.' So we *do* have the ability to control our weight. Positive Shrinking will show you how to bring this control to bear on being the weight you've been waiting to be ... starting *now*.

HOW IS IT DONE?

The system trains you to eradicate, very quickly, the emotional drivers that cause you to over-indulge. You will learn how to:

- deflate the anxieties that cause emotional (comfort) eating
- kill cravings quickly and permanently
- utilize simple formulae for *when* you eat

- stop the excuses and 'just do it'

- determine which foods are OK for you and those to which you are sensitive

- employ the FIT method (**F**ocus–**I**ntention–**T**enacity)

- and much more …

The method is explained in 'parable' style – employing a story of someone who has achieved her goals by using Positive Shrinking. It is in a style and setting which I hope most readers will be able to relate to.

WHAT IF?

What if Positive Shrinking has most of the answers you've been seeking and you use it, get results, maintain the results and tell others how you did it? What if this book became a worldwide bestseller and saved many others from being overweight (with all the emotional and clinical problems and issues that go with it)? Would there be value in that … or not? What if you became a part of that movement?

Wouldn't that be good?

FOREWORD

There is a revolution happening right now!

The world's preferred way of losing weight has been to diet; however, the overwhelming scientific research has shown that 50 years of dieting have actually made a large proportion of people in the Western world overweight. This irony would be laughable if were not so sad. By the late 20th century, many thousands of people had become overweight after starving themselves on diets.

People are now becoming aware that diets work for hardly anyone, and more and more researchers are discovering that weight gain and weight loss are really about human behaviour, rather than food.

Kevin Laye is an excellent therapist and has been one of the key people working with me at my live events in my quest to help the world lose weight easily. We have both studied people who are overweight and people who are naturally thin; we have heard many different stories and worked with plenty of 'hopeless cases'.

This book is the product of many years of research, not done in a laboratory, but in the real world.

Kevin has his own unique approach to weight loss. However, we both come from the same school of thought: weight loss is not so much about food, but really about the way people think and act around food.

When it comes to learning, some people like to read straightforward instructions; some people prefer stories; some like a mixture of both. That's why this book is so helpful to anyone wanting to lose weight and keep it off. The simple, user-friendly approach makes it possible to transform your relationship with food and the way you think and feel about yourself for ever!

Paul McKenna

ACKNOWLEDGEMENTS

Now, before I begin with my list of acknowledge-ments, I would like to state that this book would not have been possible without everything I have learned from my friends and mentors. This is not my work; it is a composite of everything I have learned from some truly amazing people. My task is to represent it to you, in what I can only hope is both an educational and entertaining narrative. With this in mind, I say thanks to the following:

Brian McCutcheon, the fireman whose passion and congruence drove me to finish this work. Thanks for pushing me to do this. Nag, nag, nag …

Martin Sterling, aka Mr Black, for the title and your wit, humour and support. Be well in heaven my friend.

Paul McKenna, a great friend, a mentor and 'the' someone who has done much more than anyone I know to help people enable themselves to take control of their weight issues with his outstanding work. Thanks, bro … for everything.

Michael Neill, the most congruent trainer I know … you are 'exactly what it says on the tin' … you teach me so much by just being you.

Richard Bandler, genius and co-creator of the field of Neuro Linguistic Programming.

Roger Callahan, creator of Thought Field Therapy, and in possession of the most inventive mind I have ever had the pleasure of experiencing, a genius, a mentor and the most giving soul I know … If God sent a gift for us to heal pain and suffering, then we have Roger to thank for discovering it and sharing it so willingly with the world. Love you so much, Roger. Thank you.

William Shakespeare, who wrote the original diet question: 'Tubby or not Tubby? … Fat is the question' … Sorry, I couldn't resist. ☺

I also acknowledge my family, all my students, friends and clients; in fact everyone I have ever met in my life, for in some way, no matter how small, you have made some communication with me and I have learned everything I have ever learned (good and bad) from you.

The final thanks must go to everyone who reads this book and uses it to change the way they do what they do with life. Thank you for trusting me to be your guide on this interesting journey. I applaud your faith in me, but applaud even louder your faith in yourself. Oh, and Nike for the inspirational phrase, 'Just do it!'

Now, let's 'weight no more' as we get ready for some Positive Shrinking!

LIST OF ILLUSTRATIONS

Figure 1. *The Psychological Reversal (PR) Triangle and Craving-busting Tapping Sequences*

Figure 2. *The Yes/No Technique*

Figure 3. *The Finger and Thumb 'Sticky' Technique*

Figures 4 and 5. *Eye Relaxation Rub Technique*

Figure 6. *Eating a PIE ... Positive Imagery Exercise*

1

HOW TO CONTROL EMOTIONAL AND COMFORT EATING

Jo sat back and rested in the hot tub, closing her eyes and letting the warmth of the water be absorbed into her skin. Her mind drifted into a fantasy of sitting in her own private hot tub on the veranda of a water bungalow overlooking the Indian Ocean as she relaxed on her dream holiday in the Maldives. In her dream she wore a very elegant turquoise bikini, size 12. She could feel just how good it could feel … 'Mmmmm, nice,' she thought.

C-R-E-A-K – the door opened and in walked one of the spa staff, with a handful of towels. Jo came back to reality and shifted herself in the hot tub as her senses noted straight away that she was not wearing a size-12 turquoise bikini, but the large black one-piece she had had for some time now. Well, black is slimming, so they say, and why buy a new one when this one is OK? Jo smiled a forced smile as she caught the eye of the member of staff, and answered 'Yes, fine thank you,' when she was asked if she was OK. 'I am just waiting for my friend Sam to arrive,' she added.

Jo and Sam had been friends since school, and although they now lived quite some distance apart they still kept in contact with phone calls, birthday cards, etc. And one thing they had done every year for the last ten was to meet up for a weekend of pampering and 'girly' time at a spa resort in the UK. This was their 11th time, and Jo was really looking forward to seeing her friend to exchange news and have fun and just have a big hug. It was great to let off steam with a friend who understood her; they had both gone down similar life paths: early career, marriage and kids, the usual stuff. 'Elevator living', they called it, full of ups and downs but getting where you wanted most of the time. This weekend they would, no doubt, as usual, spend a large part of the time discussing the latest diets and fashion tips for the more 'well covered' woman. No doubt, also, each would testify that *this* would be the year when they would 'sort things out' for themselves fitness- and weight-wise, knowing really that life would take over and they wouldn't. Well, the fantasy – like all fantasies – was nice.

'Oops, getting a bit poached,' Jo thought as she lifted herself from the hot tub and put on her white towelling dressing gown supplied by the spa. 'Never as fluffy or as big as you would like them to be,' she mused as she pulled the belt around her and stepped through the door, noting the 'creak' as she did so. 'Maintenance needed there,' she thought. All the external glamour of the place, yet it still had the odd creak here and there. Oh well … She found a chair in the 'cooling down' area, which was a huge Victorian-style conservatory giving views over the beautifully kept grounds, and as she sank back into it, picked up a magazine full of fashion tips, exercise plans and the latest 'amazing' diet that would transform your life for ever. 'Yeah, right,' she said to herself, knowing she would read it anyway, just in case.

As Jo was fully absorbed in an article on the benefits of miso soup, she heard the sound of a car pulling up. 'Great, Sam is here,' Jo thought, going to the French windows to have a look. Then the car door opened and out stepped a woman in a cream fitted suit. Jo knew as soon as she saw her that she was mistaken; this woman was way too slim to be Sam. So she returned back to the joys of the miso soup 'energizer' plan.

Having read and digested the miso soup article, Jo was now looking at an advert for an 'abdominizer' machine that promised amazing results – 'lose both pounds and inches within weeks,' the ad proclaimed. She already owned a clone of the 'abdominizer', but nonetheless continued to read every word of the advert … just in case. As Jo got to the testimonials part of the advert, the door to the conservatory opened and in walked the woman in the cream suit. Jo recognized her instantly as the woman who'd stepped out of the car earlier; what took a fraction of a second longer to realize was that it was indeed her friend Sam.

'Hi, you,' said Sam, smiling down at her friend. 'Traffic,' she added with a shrug, like this comment would explain everything to her friend, who was looking at her as if she were looking at some alien body-snatcher version of her friend. 'Hi to you, too,' replied Jo. 'My god, you look amazing.' 'Thank you,' said Sam. 'I feel it. Wanna hug?' she added as she leaned over to hug her friend with that real warmth and affection usually found only between lifelong friends. No fake air kisses here, but a real squeeze of welcome that says 'I've missed you' more than any words ever could.

When the hug broke Jo had to take another double-take at her friend, especially as she had noted that the hug, though full of affection, felt different, maybe not quite as big (literally). Then that thought balloon popped and out came the only question that could be asked when confronted with the image in front of her: **'When?'** Followed quickly by **'How?'**

'Well, let me get settled and I will divulge all to you. I'm going to get changed and join you. Will you order us some water and a pot of tea, please? Be back in ten.' 'OK,' said Jo as she watched her friend head back to the reception area.

Jo duly ordered the drinks and, as they were being delivered, Sam entered the room in her dressing gown, which seemed to fit her very well and looked somehow fluffier, too. 'I am amazed,' said Jo, 'at the way you look. What size are you now? A 12?'

'Depends where I shop,' laughed Sam. 'Mostly a ten, but in some shops I am a 12 – but I never do the measurement thing now. I have learned it's more important to go on how you feel.'

'So when you said before you'd be back in ten you meant it literally,' laughed Jo. 'So when did all this start and why haven't you mentioned it before now to me when we've spoken on the phone?'

'I guess it began after our weekend last year. I decided I was kind of sick and tired of being sick and tired, and I knew I needed to do something about it. I knew that, like you, I had done dieting to death and felt no better, and in fact often felt worse with the feelings of guilt and failure, which I fed with more things to feel guilty about as a perverse form of comfort. I knew I needed to do something different, so I found myself a system that I knew I could stick to, and that gave me the freedom I needed to enable me to control how I looked. It took a while, but eventually I adopted a methodology called **Positive Shrinking**. It is simple and effective, but like anything else, you have to work with the system for the system to work. No excuses; just do it. Well, I did it and the results are right here in front of you to see and for me to feel – and I feel good; better than I have felt in a long time. And it's not just the weight thing. I feel amazing in so many ways. Now, as to why I didn't tell you before … well, I know that every year we discuss how we want to be but had never got there because life kind of got in the way, and I also knew that I had to do this for myself and by myself for me and only me. I also thought that once I had done it, I could, if you wanted me to, teach you everything I had learned so you can do it, too. Question is, you interested or not?'

'Mmmmm, let me see,' said Jo, looking up to the right and drumming her fingers on her chin. 'Der, of *course* I want to know … everything please … *now*.' Jo laughed as Sam echoed her laugh, nodded and agreed, 'OK, then, let's just do it.'

'I was curious,' Sam began. 'I was looking at the diet industry and the thought hit me square in the face: If diets worked, then why are there so many of them? There are some 2,000 to 3,000 of them. The answer was they *do* work for a limited few, but for most they don't. So then I thought, why don't they work for those they don't work for? And the answers to that were:

- denial of the things you crave, making you want them even more

- failure to address the 'need to feed'

- history of diets not working before

- no psychological input

- boring, boring, boring

- costs.

'Bottom line is "You cannot **live** on a **die**t for your whole life" – and why should you when you no longer need to? So I made a conscious decision to look for any and all alternatives to a diet to enable me to be the person I knew I could be.

'I also realized that I was overweight and it was my fault. I heard a question asked once, which was **"When did you last eat something by accident?"** And of course the answer is "Never", which brings up the question "So why do I eat when I am not hungry?" My answers were:

- feeding the need (**the void** – the negative emotions)

- habit ... when I am fed up I get *'fed up'*

- temporary feeling of satisfaction

- wanting things I knew I shouldn't have – those "sins" (according to my diet plan).

'So obviously I needed some control over my "emotional eating" or "comfort eating". The solution I found came in the form of Thought Field Therapy. I read a book by Dr Roger Callahan called *Tapping the Healer Within,* and found it was full of techniques I could use to overcome negative emotions – especially the ones that made me feel bad enough to want to feed the void that negative emotions created in me ...'

'Sounds amazing,' Jo said. 'So how does it work?'

Sam smiled, 'Let me demonstrate it to you right now ... ready?'

'Sure,' Jo said. 'Let's just do it.'

Sam turned her chair to face Jo, and began:

'This may look a little strange, but you have to trust me because this works so well when you do it. What we are going to do is use some acupuncture points on the body. By tapping them in a certain sequence, we can negate the emotional "overwhelms" that we have and that can cause us to comfort eat.

'Basically, if you think of yourself as a computer and the overeating as a virus, you tap on your body pretty much like you would tap on a keyboard to enter the correct code or sequence to knock out the virus. The same is done by tapping on these acupuncture points in the correct sequence – and it works for most people on most things most of the time.

'So, now,' Sam continued, 'think of something that causes you some stress right now and grade it on a scale of one to ten, with ten being the most stressed and one being the least … have you got something?'

Jo scanned with her eyes for a moment, then said, 'Oh yes, I have something that is currently about an eight on that scale.'

'OK, good,' said Sam. 'Now, whilst thinking of it, tap under your eye at the top of your cheek-bone about six times … not too hard … OK, now go under your arm, either arm, about four inches down from your armpit, kind of where a bra strap would sit, and tap again six or so times. Then find the end of your collarbone, at the base of your neck, and feel the lump or "knuckle" on the end and tap about an inch underneath that too.'

Jo followed these instructions and then looked at Sam, as Sam asked 'OK, what number is it now?' Jo thought for a moment and replied, 'Er, about four … what is this? I feel all light.'

'No worries,' reassured Sam. 'That's expected. Now find the spot on the back of your hand between your little finger and ring-finger knuckle, and go back an inch and tap that continuously whilst I ask you to do some things with me. OK?' … 'Sure,' acknowledged Jo.

'Now, whilst you tap, do this:

- *Close your eyes*

- *Open your eyes*

- *Keeping your head still, look down one way and then the other*

- *Roll your eyes in a full circle one way, then the opposite way*

- *Now hum a few bars of a tune, then count one to five out loud, then hum a few bars again.'*

Jo complied, and when she had finished, announced, 'I feel really stupid.'

'I know,' Sam reassured her, 'but let me ask you again: What number is the stress now?'

Jo sighed, then smiled. 'It's gone … wow, that's a cool distraction technique.'

'No, no, no,' said Sam. 'It isn't a distraction … OK, to prove my point, now we have stopped "distracting" you with the tapping, try to get it back to an eight again.'

Jo sighed again. 'Well, I can't … oh my god, I really can't!' She then proceeded to smile, and then laugh out loud. 'Wow, that's bizarre.'

'Isn't it?' Sam smiled back. 'And we can deal with cravings just as easily. Let me show you. So, Jo, do you still like chocolate?'

'Of course, too much,' Jo said, looking down at herself. 'Wish I didn't.'

'Really? Then do this. Think of your favourite chocolate and imagine eating it right now. Feel it melting in your mouth and imagine the feeling as you swallow it in its melted form … you like?'

'Mmmmm, oh yessss,' Jo responded with a beaming smile.

'Right then,' Sam broke Jo from her choccy trance. 'Do this. Tap on that collarbone point, then the spot under your eye, then the collarbone point again.' Jo did as instructed, as Sam asked, 'Now imagine eating and swallowing that same chocolate that you enjoyed a moment ago.'

Jo again went through the motions of miming eating the chocolate she loved; however, she looked at Sam with what was almost a mix of mild panic and disgust on her face. 'Ugh,' she cried, 'it gets stuck in my throat and it tastes awful. In fact, it makes me feel quite sick.'

'Well, reactions vary,' Sam answered. 'That's quite a strong one; sometimes it's just a feeling of "I don't want it right now" through to actually feeling nauseous at the thought, which it seems is how you are feeling. Kind of **lust to disgust** in a few seconds.'

'Yeah, that about sums it up,' Jo responded. 'So does that mean I can never eat chocolate again?'

'Not at all,' reassured Sam. 'It means you have the choice now as to whether you feel compelled to have chocolate again. The Positive Shrinking programme is not about telling you what you can or can't do. It is about giving you true freedom of choice as to what you decide to eat or not. If you truly and honestly follow the techniques you should never lose control over what you eat, and we have only just started. There are many more things to come that support this. Freedom around food is about to be yours, so enjoy it.'

'Seems too easy,' said Jo. 'Well,' Sam replied, 'you can always go back to the diets if you want it to be hard and not to work.' 'OK, point made,' Jo conceded. 'So what else does this tapping stuff do?' she asked. 'It seems so powerful. I have just been trying to get back that stress and I still can't, and the thing I was thinking of really bothered me before.'

'I know,' Sam replied, 'but after a while you get used to it just fixing things such as:

- stress
- anxiety
- cravings and addictions
- trauma
- obsessive thoughts
- jealousy
- pain
- phobias and fears.

'In fact, it deals with so many things. Best thing to do is what I did: research it for yourself, or even read Dr Callahan's book.

'OK,' Sam continued, 'so now we have had a few minutes, try thinking about eating some chocolate again.'

Sam looked on as Jo tried to imagine it, and indulged in a wry smile as she watched her friend's reaction. 'Cool, huh?' asked Sam. 'Not exactly the word I would use,' Jo retorted, 'but really, really weird. Like I know I should be able to, but I just really don't want to. Seems like there is no point to it, like I can't be bothered to.'

'You ever felt that way about chocolate before?' asked Sam. 'Can't honestly think of a time when I have,' Jo answered.

Sam smiled and looked at Jo before saying, 'You see, now you are able to take it or leave it. And that applies to any and all foods where you feel you don't have a choice: simply learn the sequence we did and, before you decide whether to eat a food or not, tap the sequence out. If you still feel like you can eat it, then go ahead – but if you feel like it's a "No way", kind of like you do now, then you will never have to comfort eat again. It takes only a few seconds to tap, so there is really no excuse not to just do it. Freedom can be easy.'

2

THE CAUSE-AND-EFFECT EFFECT

After finishing the tea and the water they had ordered Jo enquired, 'So what else does this Positive Shrinking process involve, then?'

'Well,' answered Sam, 'there are a whole set of techniques which are used. Some people only need just one technique, whereas others need to do the whole thing. But saying that, it is more than just a set of techniques. It's about developing a certain attitude, a mindset, to just do it.'

'Kind of mind over matter, then,' said Jo.

Sam shrugged a little, then replied, 'Actually, it's better to see it as more "mind over platter".'

Jo laughed out loud. 'That is *so* funny! Now *that* image I can do. **Mind over platter.** That's excellent … love it.'

Sam continued. 'One thing I learned as I was researching and learning about this is that everything is down to me. It is my responsibility, from what I eat to how I eat to when I stop eating to how much I exercise – and to how much control I exercise over my choices and decisions.

'It's the law of **cause and effect**. For example, if the effect I want is to be a non-smoker, I adopt the "causality" and habits of non-smokers, like not buying cigarettes and not putting them in my mouth and lighting them. I behave like a non-smoker and thus become or stay a non-smoker.

'It is the same with weight. If you want to be slim, then do what slim people do. Eat one biscuit, not the whole tin. Learn to relax around food and lighten up on the inside so you can lighten up on the outside, too. Truth is, if you want to change on the outside you have to change on the inside first. This is what understanding cause and effect allows you to do.

'Now if you adopt the cause-and-effect mentality and do the "causal" things which will give you the effect you desire, you will get the result you want. If you don't, what you'll get is all the reasons why you couldn't do it, and these are always not really reasons but more like excuses and lies that we tell ourselves, and as we lie to ourselves we cheat ourselves of the thing we desire the most. Now how crazy is that, but how many people do it? I know I have. Have you, too?'

'Yup,' said Jo. 'Too often.'

'Let's look at some of the effects of cause and effect in action, shall we?' Sam asked.

'Sure,' replied Jo. 'I'm all ears. This stuff sounds so easy, or should I say you make it sound so easy?'

'That's just it, it *is* easy if you just do it. And I am mind-reading now, but I bet you have already had a few thoughts of how it won't work for you … am I right?'

'Am I that transparent?' laughed Jo.

'No, not at all,' Sam reassured her. 'You are just experiencing the same thoughts I had when I was first learning about this stuff. All mine began with, "Ah, yes, but …" and then I had a realization: once I understood the power of cause and effect, and its effect, I realized that I had to get off my big "yes but" and do something different to get the effect I wanted, which was to wait no more to be the slim person I wanted to be. And here I am one year on, with the security of knowing I did it without using diets but by taking control of all the other stuff. I stopped eating my emotions disguised as food.'

'Wow,' remarked Jo. 'I have known you most of my life and I have never seen you so enthused about anything. It's almost hypnotic.'

Sam smiled knowingly. 'Isn't it?' she said quietly.

'Anyway,' Sam continued, 'back to the examples of cause and effect.' **If "consistently over-weight" is the effect, let's list the causes:**

- no control over a healthy eating style
- comfort foods and emotional eating
- obsession with food and types of food
- stress carried in the body
- pain, sometimes caused by being too heavy

- years of 'yo-yo' dieting

- minimal exercise ... 'too fat to be fit'

- poor self-image leading to a 'what's the point?' mentality

- lying to ourselves that it is not in our control – i.e. have no control

- other factors such as medical problems, for example a thyroid activity issue.

'All of these can be dealt with using the Positive Shrinking techniques – except for the **medical issues, which obviously you'd have to discuss with your doctor before you began doing this**. Common sense, I know,' Sam added, 'but it has to be said.' Jo nodded.

'OK, so now let's look at the effect of being consistently slim – and *its* causes. **Consistently slim people:**

- have control over their food

- have alternatives to control stress other than food and drink

- do not obsess over food and know intuitively what to eat

- do not 'diet'
- mostly, have a good self-image
- have control over their weight.

'Please note,' Sam said, 'that the slim list is smaller and the overweight list is bigger.'

'Yes,' noted Jo. 'Forty per cent smaller, by my reckoning – which is about the amount of weight loss I need to achieve to be the perfect ten that I want to be. A coincidence or not?'

Sam left the question hanging as she carried on: 'Another thing I noted as I looked into what slim people do to cause themselves to stay slim is that they never worry about food – and, let's be honest, why should we? There is an abundance of food now in many parts of the world, and certainly in most cities and towns. I would bet that within a three-minute walk or drive you could find some food source, so there really is no need to worry or obsess about ever being hungry. You know, consistently slim people seem to have an ambivalence about food, and seem intuitively to make healthier choices because of this. They also know they look fine, so they don't beat themselves up over how they look and turn to food or drink for comfort.

'Of course there are exceptions, like people with clinical issues like anorexia or body dysmorphia, but they really are the rare exception and not the rule.'

'The "intuitive eating" thing intrigues me,' remarked Jo. 'I always make bad choices in my foods, but it is usually something I like that I know is not good for me but I eat it anyway. Madness, I know, but I can't stop myself.'

'Well, you can now,' Sam said. 'Remember the tapping for the craving? If you do that you will be unable to eat things that you know you don't want to. There is no such thing as "bad" food, just a bad choice about food – and as you say, you are aware that some food is not good for you but you eat it anyway, even though you know it makes you tired or bloated. Mother Nature is so cruel sometimes. I did come across something on my research by an American doctor called Doris Rapp. You should Google it some time, it's fascinating what she has come up with. In her studies she has noted that, in general, three of our most favourite food or drink choices are bad for us – or, as she calls them, "toxic". She doesn't mean toxic as in allergic, but more of an energy toxin, making you feel less well than you normally do.

'Some signs that you have ingested or even inhaled an energy toxin are:

- feeling bloated (usually in the form of water retention)
- lethargy
- feeling irritable
- feeling tearful and hopeless
- "loser" syndrome
- tendency to procrastinate
- insomnia or poor-quality sleep
- itching skin or even the development of eczema or psoriasis
- poor bowel movement
- sticky faeces.

'If you are aware you have or do experience any of these symptoms consistently, then there's little doubt that you are the subject of a toxic overload.

Pretty awful, I know, but worth knowing,' Sam said. 'So it really is in our best interests to select foods that are OK to eat and not toxic for us.'

'Yes, but,' began Jo, till Sam cut her off with a wagging finger and a vocal 'Ah ah' as she gently shook her head.

'OK, I am suitably chastised,' laughed Jo gently as she continued. 'So how is it possible for someone to know what foods are OK and not OK to eat and not be toxic?'

'Seems difficult, doesn't it?' Sam said. 'Which, I have to say, really bothered me until someone taught me an amazing technique that told me instinctively by self-testing what was OK or not OK for me. It is a bit weird and seems kind of witch-crafty at first, and I have no idea how it works, but I just know it does. Interested?'

'Absolutely,' said Jo, with a huge grin. 'Bring it on, the weirder the better.'

'OK,' Sam said, 'but let's order lunch first.'

3

SO WHAT'S OK FOR ME TO EAT?

With lunch ordered, Sam and Jo got themselves a table to dine at and, once settled into their chairs, Jo broke the silence with, 'So if it's witch-crafty, does that mean I need to go out and buy a pointy hat and broomstick?'

'Now you're being silly,' Sam responded. 'Of course you don't.' Jo made a face of disappointment just as Sam added dryly, 'You can have my spare ones.'

Both of them laughed before Sam began again, 'OK, hun, this is a little weird, as I said, but go with me on it, OK?' Jo nodded. 'When I first learned this I was kind of sceptical, but since I have learned to trust this method and choose what's OK for me, I feel so much better and more energized, and I can't remember the last time I got any bloated feelings with food.'

'Sounds great,' Jo said. 'So spill the beans, or do I have to give you a Chinese burn like when we were kids?'

Sam frowned as if remembering the discomfort before saying, 'Well, it all started when I was at a conference and at the coffee break I saw this woman doing something odd with her finger and thumb whilst holding a fruit tea in her hand. I remember smiling at her and asking her what she was doing. "Just making sure that this tea is OK for me to drink today," she told me. "So how does that work?" I asked. "Very well," she replied with a smile, to which I responded with a smile of my own. "Sorry," she went on, "I am being a tease; would you really like to know how to do this?" "I'd love to," I said, to which she replied, "Let's find somewhere quiet, then, so I can teach you. But," she added, "There is a price if I teach you. You need to promise me to teach what I show you to anyone you get the chance to."

'I agreed, we found a quiet spot in the reception area and she spent a short while, *because that's all it takes to learn*, to teach me the most amazing thing.'

'Sold, now just show me, too,' Jo pleaded in mock frustration.

'OK, I will,' Sam agreed, 'but you need to make me the same promise I made her: you will teach everyone who wants to learn this.'

'Deal … you got it,' said Jo with a firm nod of her head.

'Then let's begin before lunch gets here,' said Sam. 'We need to stand up, though.'

Jo and Sam stood up and made some space so the technique could be demonstrated.

THE TECHNIQUE

'What we need to do is *calibrate* ourselves. We do that by standing with our feet parallel and about nine inches apart, with a straight but not rigid back, and then just look forwards.' Sam checked that Jo was in the correct posture and position, then continued, 'Now, whilst in this position, just keep repeating to yourself in your head the word "Yes" over and over again.'

Jo giggled, 'Sorry, I just had a flash of the restaurant scene from *When Harry Met Sally* pop into my mind. I'll behave … sorry.' Sam smiled; nothing changes with Jo, she thought, and let out a mock sigh as she raised her eyes to the ceiling.

'So keep saying "yes" over and over in your mind and see what happens.' Sam waited for a few moments, knowing what would happen, and smiled again as Jo said, 'Oh, I am moving forwards, how odd.'

'OK, cool, so that's the "yes" response. Now do this,' Sam instructed. 'Get into the start position and now think the word "No" or say it over and over again in your head.'

Jo complied as Sam awaited the expected reaction. 'Whoa,' yelled Jo, as she almost fell over backwards. 'What the hell is that meant to mean?'

Sam laughed as she replied, 'I would say that's a firm No reaction, Jo. Now do this: think of the word "No" again, but as you do, try to go forwards and see what happens.' As Jo did this, Sam could see from her furrowed brow that she was realizing it wasn't possible. 'I can't,' Jo confirmed. 'It, whatever it is, won't let me. It's almost like a force pushing me back. You're right, Sam, this *is* weird.'

'I know,' Sam agreed, 'but now let's try it with some specifics. Do this: stand in the neutral spot and ask yourself, either in your head or out loud, *"Is water OK for me to drink?"* and see what happens.'

Jo did as asked, and reported, 'Well, I am going forwards, so no surprise there then.'

'Now ask yourself, *"Is it OK to drink bleach?"'*

'Okey dokey,' smiled Jo in anticipation of what would happen. 'Yup, gone back,' she said. 'Good job I don't drink bleach any more,' she said, smiling.

'Try to oppose it like before,' suggested Sam.

'Can't; it feels way too weird; it won't let me. What is it? How does it work?'

'Very well, apparently,' said Sam with a broad grin that was getting broader by the second. 'Now let's test some of the more common toxins and see what results we get, OK?' asked Sam.

Jo agreed as they tested, by asking questions in the form of 'Is wheat (for example) OK for me?' and seeing the reaction of the body as a yes or no.

Jo and Sam tested the following foodstuffs. **What would happen if you tested them, too?**

- wheat
- corn
- yeast
- dairy (milk–cheese–butter–yoghurt)
- white sugar
- potatoes
- tomatoes
- garlic
- soya
- chocolate

- white wine
- red wine
- orange juice
- bananas
- melon
- deodorant
- perfume
- mouthwash
- toothpaste
- washing powder
- nicotine.

'OK, I get the foods,' said Jo, as she noted her reactions. 'But how come we asked bout the non-food stuff?'

'Well,' Sam responded, 'not only foods can be toxins, and with this method we can test just about anything. In fact, I haven't found anything I *can't* test, so far.'

'Including men?' asked Jo with a cheeky smile. 'Stop it,' Sam replied. 'Behave.'

Just then the door creaked open and in walked a member of the spa staff with a tray holding their lunch. As he placed the tray on the table, Sam and Jo sat down again. 'Mmmmm, looks yummy,' declared Jo. 'I'm looking forward to this.'

'Well, before we pounce, can we just check something, please?' asked Sam. 'Look at what you ordered and see what came up as a "No" on your toxin list.'

As Jo did a mental checklist against her lunch, her face became more and more despondent. 'Apparently half of the things I have ordered for my lunch are toxic, including the bread, the tomato and the garlic mayonnaise,' she said.

'I know,' said Sam. 'Happened to me a few times, too, and it's tough, especially when it's something I really wanted and was looking forward to.'

'So what do I do?' asked Jo kind of helplessly. 'Eat it knowing what I know, or throw it away, which is such a waste of food and of money?'

'Well, you now know it isn't "bad" food, it just isn't good food for you right now, so it depends whether you want the waste on your waist or not,' advised Sam.

'I can see this Positive Shrinking malarkey becoming expensive,' moaned Jo.

'Not at all,' Sam replied. 'You know the techniques for pre-testing the food, etc. All you have to do is just do it *before* you decide what to eat. Make it a habit. I know you said it's a waste of money, too, but where do you want the pounds – on the plate or on your hips? I can also tell you from experience that you only forget a couple of times before you just do it. If you make it easy, it becomes easy … trust me'

'Looking at the way you look now, how can I not trust you?' said Jo. 'Everything you're saying makes sense. I guess, like everyone else, I was hoping for an easy path, a magic wand, so to speak.'

'Doesn't exist,' Sam replied, shaking her head. 'All I know is that if you apply the techniques I teach you, then you can get the same results I got. I heard that Henry Ford once said,

"If you think you can do a thing or you can't do a thing, you're right."

'What do you think right now, Jo?'

'I think I *can* if I just do it,' replied Jo resolutely. 'Now can you pass me the menu, please, so I can re-order some lunch that's OK for me to eat?'

Having re-ordered a fresh lunch, Jo looked quiz-zically at Sam and said, 'Hang on a minute – you said the woman who showed you the witchy thing was doing it by rubbing her finger and thumb, not rocking backwards and forwards. Now I *am* confused!'

'Well remembered,' Sam remarked. 'I just wanted to show you the original technique first, and the alternatives once you had understood and experienced the original … so are you ready for some more weirdness?'

'In for a penny, I guess,' said Jo. 'Oh, and please, Sam, start your lunch. My re-order will take a little while to come and I bet you're hungry after the long drive.'

'Actually I *am* hungry, so I should eat,' said Sam. 'I'll explain the finger/thumb as I eat, then.'

Sam picked up her stuffed pitta bread, took a small bite and began to chew it slowly. When she had chewed it for what seemed quite a while, she swallowed and continued, 'What you need to do is rub your finger and thumb together very gently with minimal pressure, the kind of pressure you would use if you were stroking a newborn baby's cheek. That's right,' she said, as Jo gave it a try, 'Really light – and as you rub, think of the word "yes" and see how the rubbing stays smooth and friction free. Yes?'

'Yes.' replied Jo. 'It feels smooth.'

'OK, now think of the word "No" as you rub and see what happens.' Jo did so and remarked, 'Eww, it goes all sticky, with more resistance.'

'That's right,' said Sam. 'Now, just to show it isn't going sticky just due to a build-up of friction, think of the word "yes" again and see if it goes back to being smooth.'

Jo smiled as she said, 'Wow, it does. How cool is that?'

'Very,' agreed Sam. 'OK, now test it on the water and the bleach test, thinking the questions "Is it OK for me to drink water?" and "Is it OK for me to drink bleach?" and see what happens. I know, by the way, what will happen – I want you to just do it for yourself and feel it happen.'

Jo did as asked, and sat with her mouth wide open when her finger and thumb refused to move when she thought of drinking the bleach. 'My god,' she remarked, 'my finger and thumb are jammed together.' As she said this, she noted Sam taking the second bite from her pitta bread lunch. 'But isn't it just my reaction making that happen because I know water is OK and bleach isn't?'

'I thought that, too,' Sam replied. 'So, OK then, test it on the food list. In fact, even better, test it on your new lunch that is just arriving now versus the lunch that you previously ordered.'

'OK,' said Jo, 'I will' … and as she did so she noted the new lunch was, as she put it, 'safe'.

They continued with a mix of chit-chat, catching up with news on friends and families and work, alongside breaking off every so often for Jo to check something out with her new 'toys' as she put it. 'This is amazing,' she noted, as she played with the new knowledge she had acquired.

'So,' Jo began, 'so far I can take control over my feelings and the emotional eating with the tapping thing, so I will no longer need to comfort eat or overindulge as a reaction to an emotional stress. And I am also able to use the positive and negative test to determine what foods are OK for me to eat, so I don't fill my body with toxins. But that can't be all that there is, can it?'

'Depends on the person,' Sam responded. 'We are each of us unique. Now, for some people, just taking the stress load from them will allow them not to have the bad habit of comfort eating, and that may be all they need. Others will be OK by just being able not to eat toxic foods, which will be the main reason for being bloated and holding water. Others will need to do both things, and all the other techniques in the Positive Shrinking arena. That is the beauty of this method. Nothing in it can harm you or make you worse; you can only benefit from doing it, and the more you do it the more you will notice yourself shrinking on the outside but also growing in strength and determination on the inside as you see and feel the results for yourself and take notice of what others notice about you, just the way you noticed me. Yes?'

'Wow, yes,' noted Jo. 'You do seem a lot stronger and more focused than I remember you being. Kind of more self-assured and confident and relaxed – but not arrogant. I have to say I would love to be that way, too. So do you really believe if I do these techniques I will become as motivated and driven and confident as you seem to be?'

'Why not? Just do it … and find out,' replied Sam. 'What do you have to lose except what you want to lose anyway?'

Jo finished her lunch and nodded. 'OK. That was yummy, by the way. Didn't you like yours, Sam? You seemed to be picking at it – in fact you still haven't finished it. Wasn't it nice?'

'Actually it was delicious' remarked Sam, pushing her plate away. 'But I am full. Which leads me nicely into the next real thing that really makes a huge difference in how we take back control. Interested?'

'Of course I am,' Jo replied. 'I am loving this stuff.'

4

EAT LIKE A PIG ...
LOOK LIKE A PIG

'Right then,' began Sam, 'this part is both the easiest thing to do whilst, at the same time, in some ways being the hardest. But if you just do it, then it is going to make such a difference to you.'

'Fire away,' said a waiting Jo, rubbing her hands together in a comical and exaggerated anticipation.

'It's simple,' Sam continued. **'Slow down your eating speed.'** Then she fell silent.

'Is that it?' Jo questioned.

'Yup, I am afraid so. I wish it was more difficult, but it isn't' answered Sam.

'So where does the wisdom come from to support that, then?' asked Jo.

'Well, from various sources, really,' began Sam, 'but one of the most powerful examples of it is in the Paul McKenna "I can make you thin" weight-loss system. He calls it *eating consciously*, paying full attention to your food until you can reset the missing *full signal* that tells you when it's time to stop eating.

'Because of the way we eat in current times,' Sam continued, 'we pay scant attention to the food we eat or how fast we eat it – and it becomes habitual to eat this way. The upside is when we eat fast we get a rush of happy chemicals released in our brain, making us feel good, temporarily. We get addicted to that rush, so we repeat it as a behaviour over and over again, and because we do it unconsciously we are not even aware that we do it, which makes it worse as we have literally lost control.

'Let's use animals as examples. When did you last see a fat horse? Never. So why is that? Well, let's look at how a horse eats. It eats slowly, chewing its food into mulch so it is easier to digest, then it may eat a little more until it decides it doesn't need to eat any more because something inside tells it that it's full. I am sure it is also aware that there is a plentiful supply of grass and hay around, so it never worries about a food supply for when it gets hungry later. Now, all that latter part is an assumption and not something I know, but what I *do* know is I have never personally seen a fat horse or ever heard anyone say, "Oh, look at him, he is as fat as a horse." Have you?'

Jo shook her head. 'No, I never have heard anyone call anyone a fat horse. It sounds kind of a stupid thing to say.'

'Yes,' smiled Sam, 'it does, and aren't horses graceful and beautiful, even when they eat?' she asked rhetorically.

'Next let's look at pigs,' Sam continued. 'Look at how pigs eat: straight into the trough fighting for food and eating so fast and not stopping till it is all gone, and no matter where they spot food they will just eat it straight away, all of it, and they will eat pretty much anything to satisfy their hunger.

Now, how many times have you heard someone referred to as a "fat pig" or as "fat as a pig" and, be honest, how many times have you looked into a mirror and called yourself that? Don't we say the nicest things to ourselves? So that's why I use the phrase *Eat like a pig, look like a pig.*'

Jo added, 'And I notice that when we see someone eating fast in a restaurant or in fact anywhere, we will often say, "Look at him eating like a pig!" Wow, I never thought of it that way before.'

'Also' Sam added, 'when you slow down your eating you become so aware of how fast other people eat, and it isn't at all elegant. Why, you can almost see them in a trance totally defocused from the food and not even tasting it. Mind you, that's not a bad thing with some of the junk available today. I think that's why it's called fast food: if you didn't eat it fast you would never eat it at all, because you would taste what rubbish it really is.'

'Done it,' chipped in Jo. 'I have eaten junk food in the past, hoovered it down then looked at someone else eating the exact same thing I have just eaten and asked myself, "My god, how can I have just eaten that?" It makes me feel quite sick to think about it if I am being honest.'

'Another great by-product of these techniques, especially the eating slowly, is that you begin to *taste* food again. I had forgotten how good apples can taste, and a really nice well-cooked natural dinner – you know, something you cook, not just put in a microwave and await the "ping"? When you eat slowly your taste buds will reactivate and sensitize, and good food will taste good and you will no longer enjoy poor-quality food. Make sense?'

'Total sense,' Jo replied, then asked, 'So why do they call not eating anything at all *fasting*?'

'Excellent,' Sam said as she laughed out loud. 'A real secret to making this work is to make it fun and question what we have been doing to ourselves. The more we make it fun, the more we want to do it and the more we get to where we want to be. Makes you thin…k, doesn't it?'

5

FULL – STOP

'So how does this help you know when to stop eating, then?' Jo asked. 'When I was a child I was always taught by my parents to clean my plate, as anything left was a waste.'

'I know, I was too,' replied Sam, 'and you know when I look in the mirror I see I am no longer a child, I am an adult who can make my own choices so I don't have to clean the plate any more. I resigned my membership in the *clean plate society*.'

'Yes, but isn't it hard to overcome a deep pro-gramming like that?' asked Jo.

Sam smiled. 'OK, first of all, Jo, you just did a *yes, but* and that always comes before a reason or an excuse. I also know that anything that can be programmed can be reprogrammed, and as for it being hard, let me ask you how hard is it for you to keep to a diet? Counting calories, total denial of things you would love to have, the "sin" foods, the constant checking of everything. No ... No ... No ... you would never, ever get me to behave that way again. I will stick to just doing this.'

'Well, you only have to look at you to see the proof is in the pudding when you look at you now,' agreed Jo, as she giggled, realizing that maybe that wasn't the most appropriate turn of phrase.

'Thank you,' said Sam. 'I know I am passionate about this, which is why I may seem to be being a little over-enthusiastic about the Positive Shrinking techniques, but I just know what a difference it has made to my life in more ways than just the weight, and I really would love to have you have the same experience from now on. Anyway, to answer your earlier question on how your body knows when you should stop eating and leave what's left on the plate, the theory is that by eating slowly you reset the internal awareness that you are full.

'You see,' continued Sam, 'years and years of the eating-too-fast habit has allowed you to override the trigger inside that says you are full, so you've learned to ignore it and just overeat, and the more you do it the better you get at it and the more you lose control over what you eat, and the more you put on weight and the more you hate yourself for doing it, and the more you do the same thing over and over again. It really is a damaging and dangerous habit we get into, and it's time to call a *full stop* to it … now.'

'Is there any science to support this?' enquired Jo.

'Actually, yes, there is,' Sam responded. 'Scientists have found a hormone in the gut that is produced which alerts us to when we are full. The hormone is called PYY3-36, and the perverse thing is the more overweight we get, the less of this hormone is produced, so the less chance we have of being alerted that we're full. And who said Mother Nature doesn't have a sense of humour? The good news, though, is that it is fully reversible, in that the more weight we lose, the more of this hormone is produced to alert the hypothalamus (part of the brain) that we are full. This is another indicator as to why slim people stay slim. I personally have just reprogrammed myself, so now I no longer have to think about the techniques I am teaching you; I just do it.'

'Any tricks, hints or tips on how I could incorporate them into my life and make them a habit?' Jo asked.

'Of course,' Sam replied. 'What I did was use a traffic light system as it was so easy to adopt. Just like if I were in a car, when I spot a red light I come to a full stop because not doing so would be dangerous. As I ate I kept a focus on my food, which eating slowly allowed me to do, and when I got the amber light I raised my awareness ever more, so when I got the trigger that I was full I could come to a full stop … I learned to just do it.'

'Did you ever forget or mess up?' enquired Jo 'I am sure I would.'

'Of course I did,' Sam responded honestly, with a shrug of dismissal. 'And when I did, I didn't think, "Oh, I have failed, this doesn't work." I learned from it and raised my awareness for the next time. Different schools of thought offer different time-scales, but they average out at anything between

21 and 28 days to form a new habit, and in that timescale you should already have begun to notice a difference, so the motivation to continue is getting instilled daily.'

'I like the traffic light method,' said Jo. 'It's simple and very visual – and you're right: in a car you would never run a red light, and if you did by accident – and I will be honest, I have – it *does* make you more alert very quickly and you do tend to pay more attention for the remainder of the journey, so it's a great metaphor for what I need to do. Great, I know I can do that.'

'Excellent,' smiled Sam. 'I am so glad you're willing to do this. It will make such a difference to your life. Now, shall we have a swim and a steam before we carry on a little later?'

'Mmm, sounds like a plan,' said Jo, as they stood up and wandered off to the pool area.

REVISION POINTS
Positive Shrinking So Far

- Take care of emotional/comfort eating, using the tapping technique. (Tap away your cravings.)

- Adopt the causal behaviour of slim people to get the effect of slim people. (Get the result you want or give yourself the reason why you can't.)

- Determine what is OK to eat or drink using the self-test technique. (No witch's hat or broomstick required.)

- Remember, eating like a pig means you will look like a pig. (Eat like a horse eats and see if someone ever calls you a fat horse.)

- Full STOP. (See the RED light, sense the DANGER, hit the brakes and STOP).

So far Sam has taught Jo techniques for controlling what and how she eats, with no dietary advice or saying what is 'good' or 'bad'. It is important to remember that you have all the control and, if you 'just do it', then the set of techniques will work for you. If you don't, the techniques won't work for you and you'll be back to a lifetime of yo-yo dieting and all the misery that brings you. This book is all about giving you FREEDOM: the freedom never to have to diet again – to take back control of how and what you eat and to put the fun back into eating. There are no 'sins' … no 'BAD' foods, just foods that may not be good for you because they have a toxic effect on your body. Now you can identify those, you can enable yourself to make the best choices for yourself.

This book is all about YOU. Your choices … Your freedom … Your happiness … and your success to be the YOU that YOU WANT TO BE. You can do it when you *'just do it'*.

****

Jo and Sam met later in the evening for dinner, as arranged. Sam watched as Jo scrutinized the menu, selecting what was OK to eat based on what she knew from her earlier toxin test, and where there was any uncertainty using the finger/thumb test to enable her to make the correct choice for her. Jo glanced up and caught Sam gazing at her and asked, 'Am I a good student, then, Ma'am?'

'Yes, you are,' replied Sam with a smile. 'An A-plus gold-star student. Isn't it easy when you set your mind to just do it?'

'Well, it is pretty easy to do, just takes a little thought and, as you said earlier, what is there to lose except the weight I want to lose? And if it doesn't work – though I am sure it will – then I have lost nothing, so one way or another I can't lose really, can I?'

'Do you know,' laughed Sam, 'what you just said, it was almost hypnotic?'

'Mmmmm, look into my eyes,' said Jo, feigning a mad manic stare.

'I'm under,' replied Sam, as both of them cracked up laughing. 'Told you it was fun,' said Sam.

'Indeed,' Jo responded, 'and you know what I am amazed at? The stuff I would have chosen for me if I were on a diet is showing up as not good for me, and the stuff I would have expected to be an issue is showing up as OK. How bizarre is that?'

'Told you before,' confirmed Sam. 'There isn't such a thing as "bad" food, only foods that are bad for *you* – and they're not always what you thin…k, are they?'

'Well, let's order and eat then, shall we?' Jo asked. Sam nodded in agreement.

They placed their order and waited for it to be served up for them, and as they began to eat, Sam noticed Jo making a real conscious effort to slow down her eating speed and really chew and enjoy the flavours of her food. Sam did likewise with her food and they both, in synchronicity, remarked 'Delicious, mmmmm,' with Jo then adding, 'This slow eating is so good. I haven't noticed the flavours of food for such a while.'

'Wait till you eat an apple again,' said Sam. 'Amazing the flavours, especially the Pink Lady or the Fuji apple varieties … so juicy and fresh, yummy. Shame they don't have them on the menu!'

'Well, I am curious to see what it will be like when I eat the banoffee pie,' declared Jo.

'Yup, so am I' replied Sam, with a knowing smile. 'I am just going to have a nice liqueur coffee, as it does contain all the major food groups: alcohol, caffeine and fat,' she laughed.

Jo laughed back. 'Now who is being naughty?'

'*Moi,*' said Sam, defiantly. 'Guess it will have to be a French liqueur coffee, then.'

'Decadent,' Jo said, as Sam nodded enthusiastically.

The dessert and coffee were served and Jo began to work her way slowly through the banoffee pie. About a third of the way through she put down the dessert fork and said, 'I am done, totally beaten, any more and I'd be being a pig, and I really don't want another mouthful.'

'You're retuning your sensitivity pretty quickly,' said Sam. 'Any guilt about leaving it or wasting it?'

'Not at all,' Jo responded. 'In an odd way it is very empowering to know I have control over the food rather than vice versa. I mean, the pie was OK but I could have lived without it. It was an interesting test, at any rate.'

'Testing is good,' reassured Sam. 'The way to get good at anything is to practise, and the best way to practise is to practise. And Jo, you're doing great so far.'

'Thanks,' said Jo. 'I am feeling pretty good about this.'

'Let's go and sit in the lounge with the coffees,' suggested Sam. 'I'd like to tell you about a pie that you can eat as often as you like, whenever you like … interested?'

'As long as it isn't toxic,' Jo commented. 'I don't want to eat toxic food any more. I am loving knowing this stuff. Thank you so much for sharing this knowledge with me.'

'It is actually more than just knowledge,' Sam reflected. 'What we learn is knowledge; what we know is wisdom – and using that wisdom is empowerment and, most importantly, freedom.'

'Wow,' Jo said. 'You really have gone all esoteric and Zen, haven't you?' Her tone was teasing.

'I know,' agreed Sam. 'What seems to be an interesting side effect is being able to be more relaxed about everything. I think it's a combina-

tion of the tapping and the general empowerment, which you've already noticed, plus I am no
longer stressed about my looks or fashion or my
health. I just love the control it has given me over
my life. I can honestly say I am really happy, and
if something does bother me I know the Positive
Shrinking techniques will help me out. They deal
with so much more than food, you know.'

'I kind of guessed that,' Jo looked up as she continued. 'Though I have never considered calling
myself wise until now, but it's true and it actually
feels very good.'

'Right,' Sam said, as she stood up from the table.
'Let's go and have these coffees and relax as I tell
you how to eat all the pies you want.'

'More wisdom to digest, methinks,' quipped Jo.

6

EATING THE PIE (POSITIVE IMAGERY EXERCISE)

Jo and Sam retired to the lounge area and sat on the super-comfy sofa with their liqueur coffees and sighed a comfortable sigh as they viewed the fire crackling away in front of them.

'Mmmmm, this is so nice,' remarked Jo. 'Oh, yes,' agreed Sam. 'Let's chill for a few minutes before I tell you how to eat pies.' They sat in silence, that comfortable silence between friends when, although nothing is said, much is communicated.

After they had both had their fill of the coffee, Jo smiled as she said, 'Really looking forward to finding out how eating a pie will help me get slimmer.' Sam responded, 'Depends on the pie … you ready for another instalment, then?'

Jo nodded in response.

'OK,' Sam began. 'Follow what I do. Place your right hand out in front of you at about a one-o'clock position, with your open palm facing towards you. Look into your palm and project onto it an image of you exactly as you would be if nothing could fail. Done that?'

'Kind of,' responded Jo.

'Well, whatever image you have, make it even more amazing. Remember, this is fantasy; in this exercise you cannot fail, so really crank up the image. Make the pictures bright and bold, then double what you have and then double it again till your head's giving you a wow.'

After a few moments Jo responded by saying with a smile, 'Mmmmm, well I do like what I am seeing right now.'

Sam smiled, too. 'That's right, and it is in your right hand because it's the right thing for you and the right place for it to be right now. Now look right into your right hand and only there, and as you do so place your left hand at about a nine-o'clock position, again with your palm facing you. Keep looking at your right hand and, at the same time, notice your left hand with your peripheral vision out of the corner of your eye and place into that palm an image of you as you have been with everything you'd like to be able to get rid of, to leave behind if you could now. Now it's in your left hand so you can leave it, just be aware of it as you keep looking at the amazing image in your right hand, right now … that's right.

'Now slowly begin to bring your hands together in front of you as you still focus on your right hand, but be aware of your left hand, as you look into your right hand at what you want. As your hands get closer, make sure the palm of the right hand covers the back of the left hand and look through what's in the left hand as it is overwhelmed by the image in the right hand, and at that moment take in a deep breath and, as you close your eyes and exhale, pull both hands to the top of your chest and to the middle of your breastbone and immediately let go of the left hand and drop it and all it contains, because you no longer need it, and then feel and absorb everything that feels right about the image in your right hand. That's right.' Sam could see from the reaction on Jo's face that she had 'got it', her beaming smile being the biggest clue.

This made Sam smile too as she continued. 'Now absorb that image into every muscle, nerve, fibre and tissue of your body. Take it into every cell and, as you breathe in again, surround the image with your favourite colour or even a sound, and double the intensity and then, with the next breath, double it again and see how amazing you can make yourself feel. Then when you're ready, open your eyes as if you were looking at the world through the eyes of that person, and tell me how it feels.'

'Wow,' beamed Jo. 'That's awesome, that really felt amazing. What's that technique called?'

'Eating a PIE,' responded Sam. 'The PIE being a **P**ositive **I**magery **E**xercise … ready to eat another?'

'Absolutely,' Jo answered. 'It felt amazing.'

'OK,' Sam began, 'but this time you no longer need to do the left-hand part, as that's been left behind and you can focus fully on the right thing for you, so put up your right hand at one o'clock and make another image. Maybe a holiday shot this time.'

Jo repeated the exercise several times, with even more amazing images each time she did so, doubling and doubling them, finding that the imagination has no limits. 'I like PIEs,' she announced. 'Could even get addicted to them.' She smiled. 'Feeling good for no reason ... how cool is that?'

'I know,' remarked Sam. 'We can feel really bad for no reason, but forget that we can feel good for no reason, too.' Then she added, 'Time for bed, methinks. How about one for the road before we retire?'

'Sounds good to me,' agreed Jo.

'Right then,' said Sam. 'Raise your right hand to about one o'clock and see yourself having the most amazing night's sleep and being able to remember everything we have done so far, including dealing with emotional eating, the cause-and-effect effect, eating what's OK to eat, remembering to eat like a horse so no one can ever call you a pig, and the full-stop signal. Remember to be able to remember all that as you sleep and dream tonight, Close your eyes and pull that image inside you and double it, and when you're ready, be able to open your eyes only as long as you need to, to get to your bed where you can have the most restful sleep.'

With that, both Jo and Sam opened their eyes and Jo said, yawning, 'I need my bed.'

'Me too,' echoed Sam with a yawn of her own, and with that both women raised themselves from the super-comfy sofa and went to their respective rooms to sleep on all that had occurred this day.

NEXT MORNING AT BREAKFAST

Sam waved a 'Hi' at Jo as she saw her walk into the breakfast room, and Jo responded with one of those 'I'd rather be back under my quilt' looks before smiling back at her friend. Have you ever noticed that about a smile? Whenever you give someone yours, they tend to give you theirs right back.

Jo reached the table, took her seat and sighed before saying, 'I cannot tell you how deep my sleep was last night; I guess I must have needed it.'

'Tends to happen when you let go of lots of old bad habits and baggage, kind of a relief, a lighter feeling takes over you, you feel more free. Does that sound about right?' asked Sam.

'Sounds exactly right,' replied Jo. 'Feel like I have left a ton of worries behind me and yes, I do feel a lightness or less heavy or however you want to put it. I feel different and I feel better.

'Though,' added Jo, 'as I woke this morning and had a cup of tea in my room I was really tempted to indulge in the biscuits I brought with me – in case of an emergency,' she added with a laugh and a wry smile.

'So did you have any?' enquired Sam.

'No!' responded Jo, shocked.

'Why not?' asked Sam.

'Well, I didn't want to spoil this diet-plan thing we are doing,' replied Jo.

'OK,' began Sam, 'today's learnings begin now, I guess. First, we are *not* doing a diet-plan thing. Remember, diets don't work in the long term. Secondly, if you really wanted the biscuit you could have, and should have, had it as long as it was tested to be OK for you to eat – and you know how to test now, don't you?' Sam said rhetorically. 'Also, the only other thing is that it's genuine hunger and not emotional eating. If it is genuine hunger, then you should eat.'

'OK,' Jo said, 'but how do I tell the difference between genuine hunger and emotional reactions that make me eat?'

Sam replied, 'Well, the simple yardstick is if the hunger is gradual or you have not eaten for a while, then it's genuine. However, if it is a sudden impulsive need to eat it will tend to be a reaction to an emotional circumstance.'

'OK, I get it now,' said Jo. 'And I guess the more I practise noticing the difference, the easier it will get … yes?'

'Yes, it will' confirmed Sam. 'The best way to get good at something is to practise, and the best way to practise is to practise … if that makes sense.'

Jo smiled, 'Strangely, it does.' Then she asked, 'So whilst you were learning and doing this did you ever have moments when you thought it wasn't working or you didn't do the programme as you knew you should?'

'Yes,' admitted Sam openly, 'there were times when I totally sabotaged all the good work I had been doing, but once I recognized this behaviour I had the choice and therefore the control to stop it escalating and to be aware of what made the self-sabotage happen and how to deal with it … let me explain.'

7

CONTROLLING SELF-SABOTAGE

'There are a few simple techniques we can do,' began Sam, 'to keep us out of self-sabotage and focused on what we want.' Sam began to tap the side of her hand on the 'karate chop' point with the fingers of her other hand. 'And the easiest method is to do this frequently, as it keeps us out of what Dr Roger Callahan calls "PR" or "Psychological Reversal", which is the state in which we are most likely to self-sabotage. Tap with me,' suggested Sam.

'OK,' agreed Jo, getting kind of used to the weird stuff now but enjoying it nonetheless, and as she began tapping in the same way as Sam was doing, Sam said, 'Repeat the following after me:

- I want to be focused
- I can be focused
- I will be focused
- I am focused
- I'm OK.

'Now repeat on the other hand,' continued Sam, and they both repeated the exercise a couple of times until Sam said, 'OK, and now stop ... and tell me: are your hands tingling?'

'Why yes, they are,' said Jo with a surprised look on her face. 'What is that?'

'I have no idea,' laughed Sam. 'It is just something I began to play with and found it made my hands tingle. I am guessing, but I don't know, that it's some kind of energy shift. But let me ask you: how do you feel right now?'

'Kind of focused,' responded Jo, 'but more than that … erm, excited, motivated, awake … like I just want to just do it.'

'Great,' said Sam. 'That's kind of how it gets me, too, and you can do that as often as you want with no negative side effects at all. Now try and think of not doing the system and losing weight.'

Jo's eyes scanned around for a minute before she sighed gently and said, 'I can't, that doesn't seem to compute, like my mind won't allow the negative thoughts to intrude, if you know what I mean.'

'I know exactly what you mean,' nodded Sam as she continued. 'Now, another technique I have learned to use to combat self-sabotage is also used in the TFT (Thought Field Therapy) tapping, called *collarbone breathing*. Want to copy me whilst I show you how it's done?'

'Sure,' agreed Jo.

'Follow this, then,' Sam instructed. 'First, find the "knuckle" on the inner end of your collarbone where it joins the top of the breastbone. There's one on each side. Then drop your fingers down about an inch to the first soft space above the first "rib". That's the collarbone point. OK, now, place the fingertips of one of your hands – either one as you're going to do both anyway – and once you have your fingertips there begin to tap the back of the hand with the fingtertips of your other hand, between the little finger and the ring-finger knuckle. Continue to tap as you do this breathing pattern:

- Take a deep breath in and hold it for a couple of seconds

- Release half the breath and hold it for a couple of seconds

- Release all the breath and hold for a couple of seconds

- Take in half a breath and hold it for a couple of seconds

- Then breathe normally.

'Now fold your fingers and put your first knuckles where the fingertips were and, making sure your thumb does not make any contact with your skin, tap the same spot on the back of the hand and repeat the breathing exercise as you continue to tap.

'Then, once that has been done, move the knuckles of the same hand across to the other collarbone point and tap as you do the breathing.

'Once that is completed, open your hand so your fingertips are now touching the collarbone point and repeat the tapping and the breathing again.

'That's one half of the exercise done. Now repeat it on the other hand, using exactly the same hand positions, tapping and breathing till the exercise is complete.'

Once both Sam and Jo had completed this exercise, Sam asked Jo, 'How do you feel now?'

'Really relaxed, a bit spacey, but kind of energized, too,' Jo responded.

'Try to think of something negative now and get bothered by it,' suggested Sam.

Jo scanned again and then laughed as she said, 'I can't, like I don't care, sort of, I can't be bothered to be bothered about being bothered.'

Sam laughed aloud. 'What a great way to put it! That's exactly it. I actually call it the *carriage clock exercise* – you know, the old clocks with the glass dome over them, it's like the exercise puts this glass dome kind of bubble of calm around you, and although you can see out at everything you need to see, if negative stuff tries to get to you it just hits the glass and gets repelled, bounces off, it just can't get to you.'

'Perfect way to describe it' agreed Jo. 'I have been trying to think of negative issues but just can't be bothered.'

'Well, I do the collarbone breathing every morning in an almost ritualistic manner. It only takes two minutes and it gets me focused, and I just seem to have better days as a result. Not much gets to me now, and if anything is really overwhelming I can either tap it away or redo the collarbone breathing and it seems to do the trick. The bottom line is I am back in control of my emotions. I am driving my own bus,' said Sam with a firm nod.

'Driving your own bus?' Jo repeated with a little frown.

'Yes,' smiled Sam. 'Dr Richard Bandler, one of the co-creators of NLP, which is short for Neuro Linguistic Programming, wrote a book called *Using Your Brain for a Change*. In it he uses a metaphor of seeing your brain like a bus and to notice who is driving it. You see, if someone else is driving the bus, you're going to end up where *they* want to take you – and that may not be the place you really want to go or even the best place to go, and also they decide who rides on the bus with you and some of the passengers you have along may not be all that friendly or useful to you. Passengers such as guilt, anger, negativity, stress, pain, frustration, jealousy, etc., and you have to notice them as they are your companions for the ride to wherever you end up going.

'Now, if *you* take over the bus and drive it,' Sam continued, 'because you're the driver you decide who gets to ride on the bus and the destination you set for yourself, so you now have the right to kick off all the unsavoury passengers and to set the bus in the direction you choose. You can also notice as you look in the rear-view mirror as you look back on all the elements you kicked off the bus that they seem to get further and further away from you the more control you take and the more you head in the direction you choose to head off into.'

'That makes a ton of sense,' said Jo as she sat absorbing this new train (*well, bus*) of thought.

'Thinking positive is the key, which is why it's called Positive Shrinking,' said Sam. 'In fact, I have a little mantra that goes **Negative thinking will negate Positive Shrinking**.'

'I like that,' smiled Jo.

'Me too,' replied Sam, smiling back at her friend. 'And that's the kind of thing to do to stop the self-sabotage from happening. It works for most people most of the time. The thing to remember is if you fall off the wagon on the odd occasion, then just get back on it rather than beating yourself up for failing. You only really fail if you fail to continue with a system that will work for you. You really have to just do it.

'Let's finish breakfast, then,' continued Sam, 'and then I can tell you all about being FIT.'

'Can't wait,' responded Jo, pulling a fake *eek* look as she said it.

GETTING FIT

After their leisurely breakfast, Sam and Jo went to their room to get changed, and agreed to meet in the garden area so they could take a nice walk in the grounds. The weather was perfect: bright sunshine but with a crisp feel to the morning air.

Jo arrived first outside the front of the spa building and waited for Sam, drinking in the peace and quiet, and then she saw Sam and smiled inwardly at the difference in her friend, who now looked not only healthier but also calmer and more at peace. 'Serene' was the word that sprang to mind.

Sam smiled back at Jo and said, 'You seem pretty smiley.'

'No idea why,' Jo responded. 'The FIT thing you mentioned hits my *No* buttons … the idea of pushing weights around is not fun.'

'Totally agree,' said Sam. 'Yet I was, and you are, able to carry weights around all the time on our bodies, just in the form of fat.'

'Fair point,' Jo conceded, 'but it goes on gradually so you don't notice it, really.' 'That's right,' agreed

Sam, 'and when you diet you don't notice it coming off, either, so that's why people give up … they seem to expect to wake up one day and have lost a stone in the night, or become a slave to the scales, and whichever way the needle goes dictates how good or bad the day will be for them.'

'Yup, been there,' said Jo. 'Still am, I guess. It's just that it seems so hard to do, to maintain, so I get despondent almost like I can't control my weight.'

Sam replied, 'OK, let me tell you the story of a hypnotherapist called Milton Erickson. He was an amazing hypnotist who got amazing results, usually just by telling stories. Well, one client, the sister of someone whom he had treated successfully previously, went to see Dr Erickson and said she had a weight issue and couldn't control her weight, and would Dr Erickson take her on as a client and help her. Erickson agreed on the condition that she did precisely as she was instructed. The woman, desperate for help, agreed. Erickson then told her to go home and not return to see him until she had put on ten pounds in weight. The woman was distraught, but Erickson reminded her of the agreement to do precisely as instructed, so she reluctantly went away, somewhat tearfully, and returned to Erickson some weeks later, stating that she had indeed "managed" to gain the extra ten pounds as instructed – to which Erickson replied, "See? You do have control over your weight. Now let's focus on losing it."

'That's the first part of FIT,' continued Sam. '**F** for Focus. We don't lose the ability to control weight, we lose the focus or desire to control it.'

'Oh, but it is my desire to lose weight!' said Jo. 'It just doesn't seem to work.'

'Hmmm, OK,' said Sam. 'Apologies upfront for one, sounding like I am lecturing, and two, for maybe hitting you with a hurtful truth, but here goes … in fact, let me ask you something, OK?'

'OK,' said Jo, preparing for the worst.

Sam continued, 'Just suppose I asked you to run a marathon in three months' time. Would you be able to do it?'

'No way,' said Jo, laughing. 'Three years, maybe, and then it might take me the three months to complete it.'

'OK,' Sam said, 'what if I said if in three months' time you ran a marathon I would give you, cast-iron guarantee, £3 million tax free … could you run it then?'

The shift in Jo and her thinking was visible, almost tangible. 'Well, of course,' she said. 'I'd give it my very best shot.'

'So,' asked Sam. 'What has changed: the ability or the desire?'

'OK, you've got me there, but 3 million is a lot of money,' said Jo.

'Agreed,' said Sam. 'Now let's look at it another way: if your doctor told you that if you did not lose weight you would die in a year, would you lose it then?'

'Morbid thought,' said Jo, 'but again, yes I would.'

'Good answer,' Sam said with a wry smile, 'and you would pay anything to be in good health, I am sure … even the 3 million for the marathon – so why not decide *now* to invest in your health so the doctor will never have to tell you you have to make that choice? All you have to do is *focus* on what you really want. And this also covers the 'I' part of the FIT philosophy: 'Intention'. It's about focusing on the *WIIFM*: the "What's In It For Me" part of your focus on change.'

Jo responded, 'You mean how I will feel and look, etc.?'

'Precisely,' agreed Sam. 'And it's easy, really. Every time you feel you may be sabotaging your long-term goal, make a picture in your mind of how you want to look and feel, and ask yourself, *Will the behaviour I am about to do help me or hinder me in achieving that outcome?*'

'OK, got that, boss,' Jo said with a nod of the head and a chuckle. 'So best tell me what the "T" is in FIT, then.'

'Tenacity,' said Sam in a very matter-of-fact way, 'to keep going even when you fall off the wagon – and you will, just like I did quite a few times, and give in to cakes and biscuits or that extra slice of toast. It is all to easy to go, *Oh, I have failed again, I am doomed to be fat* when really you just have to say to yourself *Oops* and realize it is time to carry on as before and learn from the blip, because that's all it really is, a blip, not an excuse to admit defeat … I think it was Winston Churchill who said, **"Never, never, never never never never never quit!"**

'In fact,' continued Sam, 'think about it: Olympic athletes, to win a gold medal or achieve a personal best, have to focus on what they do and have the intention of achieving the outcome they want, and they have the tenacity to do all they can to achieve that outcome. Well, my gold medal is my health and being well and staying this way from now on … I can win, and so can you.'

'Wow,' said Jo after letting out a gasp, realizing she had been holding her breath. 'You really are fired up, aren't you? Well, that version of getting FIT I am able to do, and at least it has nothing to do with pushing weights.' Jo reconsidered her words, 'No, it *is* pushing weight, but it is pushing it off my body from now on.'

Sam smiled a huge smile and nodded in agreement with her friend. 'You got it, girl.'

Jo stopped for a moment and looked back over her shoulder at the spa building, now a long way away, and said, 'Oh, look. Look how far we have come.'

'Yup, we have,' acknowledged Sam. 'Want to go back now?'

'Erm, no,' said Jo. 'I'd like to carry on if that's OK with you.'

Sam just nodded and smiled, and a quiet voice in her mind said, 'I did it … and so can you.'

AND SO CAN YOU.

Author's Note: Trying to change something by 100% will usually lead to failure … it's too big. However, you can change a hundred things by 1%, and that's what makes the difference. *The small things make the big difference.*

My best wishes for you on your journey. Now … just do it!

APPENDIX
THE GETTING FIT EXERCISES
(No Gym Necessary)

All the exercises in this section are what have been discussed in the narrative, set out in an easy-to-read (and do) format. You want results? OK, then, just do it!

CRAVING-BUSTING TAPPING SEQUENCES

Cravings mask anxieties, and because anxieties can be complex we have a few variations for the craving-busting sequences. If one is not successful, then try another.

Always do the Psychological Reversal (PR) Triangle prior to doing any sequence.

The PR Triangle

Tap the 'karate chop' bit on the side of your hand (see Figure 1, page 88), point and say:

I want to be …..............…….. (slim/thin/fit/healthy or whatever you choose to say)

I can be …....................………

I will be …....................……….

I am ……………....................…..

I'm OK.

Tap under your nose 30 times

Tap your chin 30 times

Tap your other hand and say:

I want to feel even better

I can feel even better

I will feel even better

I am going to feel even better

I'm OK

I'm more than OK.

Then do the appropriate craving sequence (there are three).

Tapping Chart

(use these appropriate points to tap cravings away)

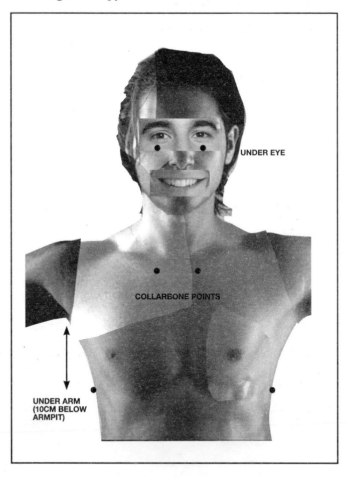

Craving Sequence 1

(See page 88 for where to tap.)

Tap, using two fingertips, ten times on each spot:

- Collarbone point (inner end under the knuckle)

- Under the eye

- Collarbone point (inner end under the knuckle).

Tap the back of your hand near your little-finger knuckle continuously:

- Close your eyes

- Open your eyes

- Look down to the left

- Look down to the right

- Roll your eyes one way, then the other

- Hum a few bars of 'Happy Birthday'

- Count one to five aloud

- Hum a few bars again.

Tap the collarbone point (inner end under the knuckle).

Tap under your eye.

Tap the collarbone point (inner end under the knuckle).

Craving Sequence 2

Tap, using two fingertips, ten times on each spot:

- Under the eye
- Under the arm on the side of the body four inches down
- Collarbone point (inner end under the knuckle).

Tap the back of your hand near your little finger knuckle continuously:

- Close your eyes
- Open your eyes
- Look down to the left
- Look down to the right
- Roll your eyes one way, then the other

- Hum a few bars of 'Happy Birthday'
- Count one to five aloud
- Hum a few bars again.

Tap under your eye.

Tap under your arm on the side of your body, four inches down.

Tap the collarbone point (inner end under the knuckle).

Craving Sequence 3

Tap, using two fingertips, ten times on each spot:

- Under the eye
- Collarbone point (inner end under the knuckle)
- Under the arm on the side of the body four inches down
- Collarbone point (inner end under the knuckle).

Tap the back of your hand by your little finger knuckle continuously:

- Close your eyes
- Open your eyes
- Look down to the left
- Look down to the right
- Roll your eyes one way, then the other
- Hum a few bars of happy birthday
- Count one to five aloud
- Hum a few bars again.

Tap under your eye.

Tap your collarbone point (inner end under the knuckle).

Tap under your arm on the side of your body, four inches down.

Tap the collarbone point (inner end under the knuckle).

Pain Sequence

- Tap the spot (between the little finger and ring-finger knuckle on the back of your hand) 50 times

- Tap the collarbone point ten times

- Tap the back of your hand by your little finger knuckle continuously

- Close your eyes

- Open your eyes

- Look down to the left

- Look down to the right

- Roll your eyes one way, then the other

- Hum a few bars of 'Happy Birthday'

- Count one to five aloud

- Hum a few bars again

- Tap the spot (between little finger and ring-finger knuckle on the back of the hand) 50 times

- Tap the collarbone point ten times

THE YES/NO TECHNIQUE

To test if something is OK for you, stand with your feet nine inches apart and parallel. To calibrate, think of the word 'Yes' – your body will usually move forwards. Then think the word 'No'; the body usually moves backwards. Sometimes it does the opposite, so take that as your calibration for the day.

Then ask if something is OK for you, for example 'Is wheat OK for me?' Notice which way your body moves to give you your answer. All questions asked must have a 'Yes' or 'No' response, otherwise you will get confused responses.

The belief system behind this is that the body intrinsically knows what is OK or not OK for it to ingest or even inhale.

The Yes/No Technique

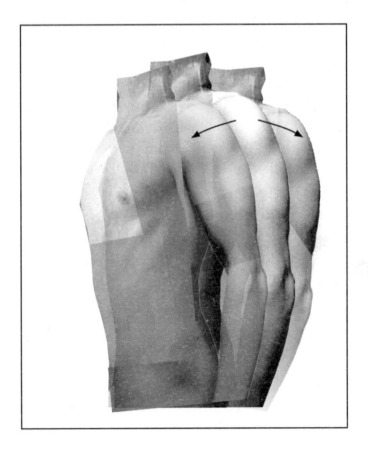

Finger and Thumb 'Sticky' Technique

An alternate method is the finger and thumb technique. Rub your first finger and thumb together very gently. Again, think 'Yes' and it should feel smooth, whilst thinking 'No' will make it go rougher or feel 'different' in some noticeable way. If you have trouble with the finger and thumb exercise, then use a credit card and rub it gently on the smooth side. 'Yes' will be easy and 'No' will have more friction and feel 'sticky'.

You can test pretty much anything utilizing this method.

Finger and Thumb 'Sticky' Technique

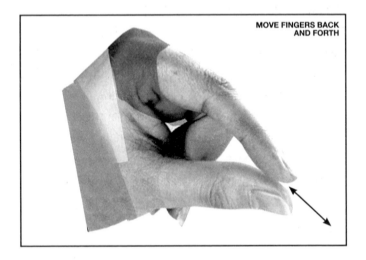

MOVE FINGERS BACK
AND FORTH

DEALING WITH SELF-SABOTAGE

For those self-sabotage feelings, first do the PR Triangle (see page 86) and also the Collarbone Breathing daily.

It is wise to do collarbone breathing daily, and best first thing in the morning.

Collarbone Breathing

First find the 'knuckle' on the inner end of your collarbone where it joins the top of the breastbone. There's one on each side. Then drop your fingers down about an inch to the first soft space above the first 'rib'. That's the collarbone point. OK now place the fingertips of one hand – either one as you're going to do both anyway – and once you have your fingertips there, begin to tap the back of the hand with the fingertips of the other hand, tapping between the little finger and ring-finger knuckle. Continue to tap as you do this breathing pattern:

- **Take a deep breath in and hold it for a couple of seconds**

- Release half the breath and hold for a couple of seconds

- Release all the breath and hold for a couple of seconds

- Take in half a breath and hold it for a couple of seconds

- Then breathe normally.

Now fold your fingers and put your first knuckles where your fingertips were and, making sure your thumb does not make any contact with your skin, tap the same spot on the back of the hand and repeat the breathing exercise as you continue to tap.

Once that has been done, move the knuckles of the same hand across to the other collarbone point and tap as you do the breathing.

Once that is completed, open your hand so your fingertips are now touching the collarbone point and repeat the tapping and the breathing again.

That's one half of the exercise done. Now repeat it on the other hand, using exactly the same hand positions, tapping and breathing till the exercise is complete.

EYE RELAXATION RUB TECHNIQUE

This simple technique allows you to get instant stress relief from any worrying thoughts or obsessive cravings around food, too. Some people just use this one technique to control anxiety and food cravings. So simple.

- Use your index finger to rub along the bone under your eye till you find the 'V' indentation.

- Place a finger each side of the 'V'.

- Massage in a small circle one way, then the other.

- Massage it back the other way, but with twice the pressure.

- Massage back the other way, but take the pressure off.

Eye Relaxation Rub Technique

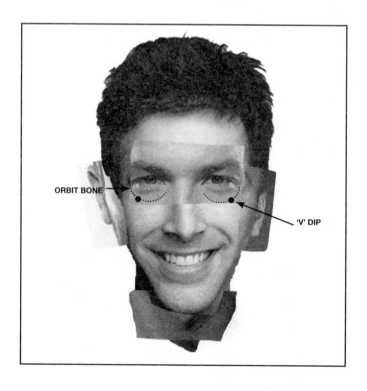

Eye Relaxation Rub Technique

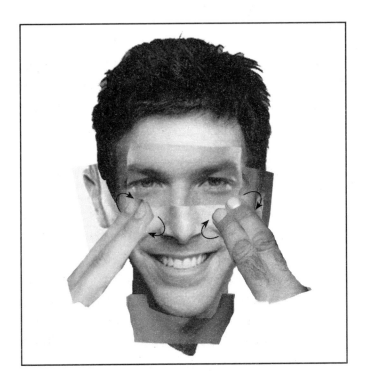

EATING A PIE ...
POSITIVE IMAGERY
EXERCISE

Raise your right hand up and to the right of you, so you are looking up at it ... Look into your palm and create a compelling image of what you want to be like, assuming that nothing can fail.

Then double the intensity of the picture and brighten it. Then double it again and again ... when it looks amazing – and only then – take a deep breath in and, as you exhale, pull the image into your chest and absorb it through your heart. Then, as you breathe in, intensify the image and, as you exhale, drive the feeling through your body into every cell, muscle, nerve, fibre and tissue until you are saturated with the good feeling. Then repeat with another good image.

Do this as often as you like ... after all, who can ever have enough good feelings?

Eating a P.I.E. ...
Positive Imagery Exercise

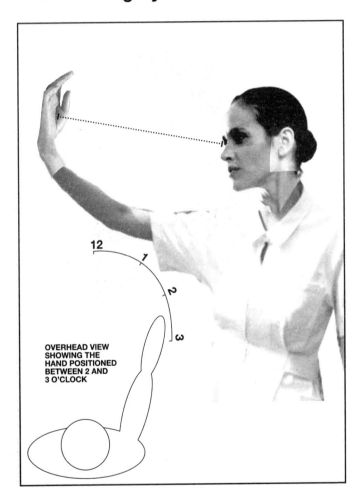

**OVERHEAD VIEW
SHOWING THE
HAND POSITIONED
BETWEEN 2 AND
3 O'CLOCK**

12
1
2
3

Eating a P.I.E. ...
Positive Imagery Exercise

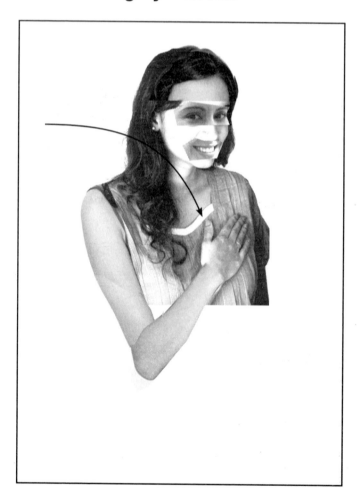

FURTHER READING AND RESOURCES

Richard Bach, *Jonathan Livingston Seagull* (MacMillan, 1973)

Dr Richard Bandler, *Using Your Brain for a Change* (Real People Press, 1985)

Dr Roger Callahan, *Tapping the Healer Within* (Piatkus, 2001)

Paul McKenna, *I Can Make You Thin* (Bantam Press, 2007)

Michael Neill, *You Can Have What You Want* (Hay House, 2009)

SUGGESTED WEBSITES

www.kevinlaye.co.uk
www.positiveshrinking.com
www.drrapp.com
www.paulmckenna.com
www.inmindtraining.com

TESTIMONIAL

Before I met Kevin Laye, I spent years on the yo-yo diet treadmill; I would lose weight and then soon pile it back on, year after year. As soon as I achieved any weight-loss goal, I lost momentum and started to put weight steadily back on. I found I had a tremendous ability to self-sabotage my weight-loss efforts, give in to my cravings and lose control of my eating. As a consequence, my weight slowly crept up, each time a little more. I felt constantly ashamed, out of control, negative and down, with an overwhelming sense of despair. The problem got worse once I had my children and my weight just kept on increasing after that! At my heaviest, I was a dress size 22 and topped the scales at 15st 5lbs. I'm only 5'2" so I looked absolutely gargantuan! I felt constantly tired, ill, uncomfortable and utterly miserable. Once, a friend of my son's called me a fat cow in front of him. I was mortified! The more miserable I became, the more I ate. I was out of control with no way of knowing how to stop. I was put on medication to treat my very high blood pressure. I was suffering from panic attacks and couldn't walk upstairs without severely losing my breath! I felt so utterly miserable that I was crying out for antidepressants.

Six years ago, I started exercising with the help of a personal trainer. However, that wasn't enough. Then I heard about Kevin and promptly made an appointment to see him at his Harley Street office. The rest is history! I gained control over my eating and today I maintain my weight between 10 stone and 10st 5lbs and wear a UK size 10. I am off all medication and my blood pressure is normal. With Kevin's help I have transformed myself and my life!

It has impacted my life to such an extent that I set up my own life coaching company: www. successfullifecoaching.co.uk. Before, I could hardly drag myself out of bed, let alone re-train myself and set up my own business. I use the

Positive Shrinking techniques to help my friends and clients gain control over their own weight demons, with great success! I now even run 10K races! My whole family has benefitted as a result. I enjoy them to the fullest and feel I am a good role model for my children rather than a total embarrassment. I am the happiest I have ever been in my life. My marriage is the best it has ever been, too! My husband and I have a passionate, very close and intimate relationship. At my heaviest our marriage was in shreds because I was so miserable!

Kevin taught me invaluable skills, which are all in this book. The Positive Shrinking techniques are now a habitual part of my daily life. I have been able to achieve and maintain my healthy weight and fitness for the past four years. For the first time in my life, I am completely happy with myself, not because I am perfect but because I am in control of my eating and my life!

Positive Shrinking techniques showed how my focus had been on losing weight and on what I *didn't* want. This placed my mind's attention on 'not being fat' or on 'losing something', instead of on a *desired* outcome. After all, we all get more of what we focus on. Not only that, once one achieves a goal, the brain can sometimes switch off and say 'Right, done!' and lose focus or momentum. This is the point at which one starts to pile the pounds back on. Focusing on achieving *and* maintaining a healthy body gives us a whole different and far more positive perspective. Instead of not wanting to be fat, my focus has become 'I am fit and healthy'.

Once I reframed my approach to achieving health and fitness, I understood why I self-sabotaged myself. While bearing in mind that understanding *why* one does things doesn't always lead to change, in this case it does. Positive Shrinking techniques not only explain why I self-sabotaged my weight-loss efforts, they gave me the know-how to help eliminate cravings and self-sabotaging behaviour.

Positive Shrinking is not another diet, it's a lifestyle! It gives me complete control over my eating habits and has taught me techniques to help control my mind. In the past, food and emotions controlled me. In my opinion, a weight problem is not an eating problem, it's a mental one!

I can honestly, hand-on-heart, say that I am now one of the happiest people on earth! The freedom that comes from learning techniques to help control my tendencies to self-sabotage and over-eat is nothing short of transformational, in every sense of the word! I feel I have been given a new lease of life and the chance to make up for all those years I spent in fat despair!

Those who only knew me before I came across Kevin's techniques often don't recognise me at first. The change has been not only physical but, more importantly, mental.

I would recommend anyone who reads this book to embrace it. It is fast and easy to read. The system works. Just do it! *Positive Shrinking* is full of hidden gems and words of wisdom, and is revolutionary in its approach! And it could transform your life!

I find it very painful to see old pictures of myself so incredibly miserable inside, out of control and overweight. I only wish I had come across these techniques sooner.

Caroline Rougemont

NOTES

NOTES

NOTES

NOTES

NOTES

NOTES

NOTES

Hay House Titles of Related Interest

Be Happy,
by Robert Holden

Calm,
by Denise Marek

Men, Money and Chocolate,
by Menna van Praag

Mindless Eating,
by Brian Wansink

You Can Have What You Want,
by Michael Neill

Your Health Is Your Wealth,
by Jacqueline Harvey

JOIN THE HAY HOUSE FAMILY

As the leading self-help, mind, body and spirit publisher in the UK, we'd like to welcome you to our family so that you can enjoy all the benefits our website has to offer.

 EXTRACTS from a selection of your favourite author titles

 COMPETITIONS, PRIZES & SPECIAL OFFERS Win extracts, money off, downloads and so much more

 LISTEN to a range of radio interviews and our latest audio publications

 CELEBRATE YOUR BIRTHDAY An inspiring gift will be sent your way

 LATEST NEWS Keep up with the latest news from and about our authors

 ATTEND OUR AUTHOR EVENTS Be the first to hear about our author events

 iPHONE APPS Download your favourite app for your iPhone

 HAY HOUSE INFORMATION Ask us anything, all enquiries answered

join us online at **www.hayhouse.co.uk**

 292B Kensal Road, London W10 5BE
T: 020 8962 1230 E: info@hayhouse.co.uk

We hope you enjoyed this Hay House book.
If you would like to receive a free catalogue featuring additional
Hay House books and products, or if you would like information
about the Hay Foundation, please contact:

Hay House UK Ltd
292B Kensal Road • London W10 5BE
Tel: (44) 20 8962 1230; Fax: (44) 20 8962 1239
www.hayhouse.co.uk

***

Published and distributed in the United States of America by:
Hay House, Inc. • PO Box 5100 • Carlsbad, CA 92018-5100
Tel: (1) 760 431 7695 or (1) 800 654 5126;
Fax: (1) 760 431 6948 or (1) 800 650 5115
www.hayhouse.com

***

Published and distributed in Australia by:
Hay House Australia Ltd • 18/36 Ralph Street • Alexandria, NSW 2015
Tel: (61) 2 9669 4299, Fax: (61) 2 9669 4144
www.hayhouse.com.au

***

Published and distributed in the Republic of South Africa by:
Hay House SA (Pty) Ltd • PO Box 990 • Witkoppen 2068
Tel/Fax: (27) 11 467 8904
www.hayhouse.co.za

***

Published and distributed in India by:
Hay House Publishers India • Muskaan Complex • Plot No.3
B-2• Vasant Kunj • New Delhi - 110 070
Tel: (91) 11 41761620; Fax: (91) 11 41761630
www.hayhouse.co.in

***

Distributed in Canada by:
Raincoast • 9050 Shaughnessy St • Vancouver, BC V6P 6E5
Tel: (1) 604 323 7100
Fax: (1) 604 323 2600

***

Sign up via the Hay House UK website to receive the Hay House
online newsletter and stay informed about what's going on with your
favourite authors. You'll receive bimonthly announcements
about discounts and offers, special events, product highlights,
free excerpts, giveaways, and more!
www.hayhouse.co.uk